I Can Heal My Family

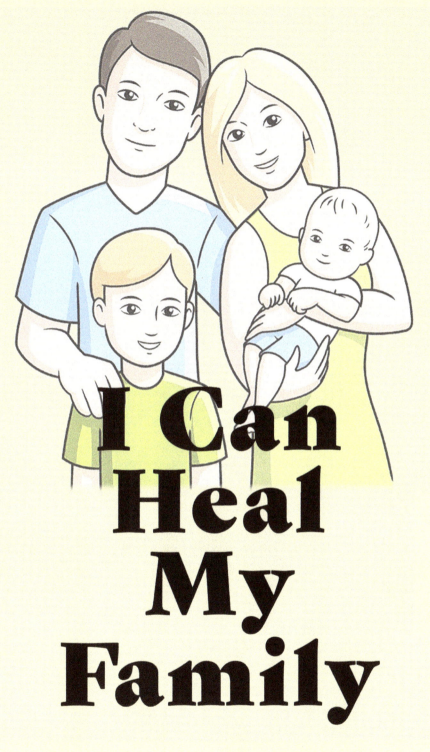

I Can Heal My Family

Kory L. Wilson

XULON PRESS

Xulon Press
555 Winderley Pl, Suite 225
Maitland, FL 32751
407.339.4217
www.xulonpress.com

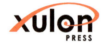

© 2024 by Kory L. Wilson

All rights reserved solely by the author. The author guarantees all contents are original and do not infringe upon the legal rights of any other person or work. No part of this book may be reproduced in any form without the permission of the author.

Due to the changing nature of the Internet, if there are any web addresses, links, or URLs included in this manuscript, these may have been altered and may no longer be accessible. The views and opinions shared in this book belong solely to the author and do not necessarily reflect those of the publisher. The publisher therefore disclaims responsibility for the views or opinions expressed within the work.

It is not legal to reproduce, duplicate, or transmit any part of this document in either electronic means or printed format. Recording of this publication is strictly prohibited.

Unless otherwise indicated, Scripture quotations taken from the Holy Bible, New International Version (NIV). Copyright © 1973, 1978, 1984, 2011 by Biblica, Inc.™. Used by permission. All rights reserved.

Paperback ISBN-13: 979-8-86850-453-2
eBook ISBN-13: 979-8-86850-454-9

TABLE OF CONTENTS

Introduction.. vii

PART 1: MY MEDICINE TOOLBOX 1

   1.   Honey Helps 1

   2.   Use Lemon Water 2

   3.   Use Grated Frozen Lemon Peel 3

   4.   Smoothie Recipes 4

   5.   Eat Walnuts 6

PART 2: SOMEONE IN MY FAMILY NEEDS HELP 7

   1.   Someone got attacked by a bug 7

   2.   Someone Has a Sunburn 8

   3.   Someone I Love Has Cancer 9

   4.   Someone Has a Cold 11

   5.   Someone Has the Flu 14

   6.   Someone Thinks They Are Going to Throw Up 15

        b.   Someone Has a Headache 16

        c.   Someone Has a Toothache 17

Introduction

As a young boy I lost my mother to cancer. Because of that experience, in my later years, I became passionate about finding cures for illnesses. I felt helpless wanting to help my mother when she came home from the hospital but could only provide love to her. This book reflects my encouragement to children of all ages that they can help to heal their family in a healthy, holistic way.

Later in life I raced bicycles semi-professionally and my health became very important to me. I collected and researched various remedies for illnesses as I did not have time to be ill nor did I have the resources to visit the doctor.

This is a collection of simple to use remedies that I hope kids can use in their desire to help heal their family.

NOTE: I am not a doctor. None of these remedies should be considered prescriptions. All content found in the book is used at your own risk.

And God is able to bless you abundantly, so that in all things at all times, having all that you need, you will abound in every good work.

> 2 Corinthians 9:8 NIV

PART 1:
MY MEDICINE TOOLBOX

1. Honey Helps

How can I use honey to help my family?

1. SLEEP: ⅓ teaspoon (tsp.) Nutmeg + 1 tablespoon (tbsp.) honey + 1 cup warm water at bedtime
2. TOOTHACHE: 1 teaspoon (tsp.) cinnamon or 4 drops cinnamon essential oil + 1 teaspoon (tsp.) honey + 1 cup warm water. Hold mixture in mouth and spit after 1-minute. Use 4 times a day
3. COUGH: ½ cup or 3 tablespoon (tbsp.) honey + 1 medium ginger root or 2 tsp. ginger. Use 3 times a day
4. SORE THROAT: 1 cup warm water + ½ teaspoon (tsp.) lemon juice or ½ teaspoon (tsp.) licorice + 1 tablespoon (tbsp.) honey. Use 3 times a day
5. SINUS: 1 tablespoon (tbsp.) honey + 1 cup warm water + 1 teaspoon (tsp.) ginger juice. Use 3 time a day
6. WEIGHT LOSS: 1 cup warm water + 1 teaspoon (tsp.) honey + ½ teaspoon (tsp.) Cinnamon after waking up in the morning.
7. COLD: 1 cup warm milk + 1 teaspoon (tsp.) honey + ¼ teaspoon (tsp.) of black pepper. Use 3 times a day
8. ACNE: 2 tsp. honey + 5 drops of tea tree oil. Apply on face as needed.

2. <u>Use Lemon Water</u>

Health Benefits:

- Someone needs help going to the bathroom.
- Someone needs to recover from exercise.
- Someone does not want a cold or flu.
- Someone is injured and has swelling.
- Someone has problems with their skin – a sunburn or they fell and skinned themselves.
- Someone is dehydrated.
- Someone wants to lose weight.

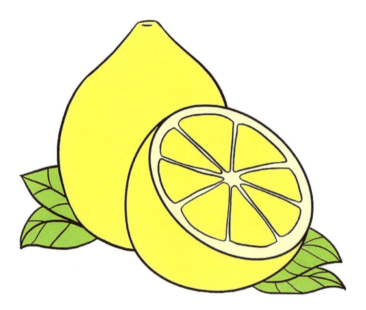

3. Use Grated Frozen Lemon Peel

Health Benefits:

- Someone has Diabetes.
- Someone wants to lose weight.
- Someone has Cancer.
- Someone does not want to get sick.

Directions:

- Freeze and grate peel.
- Sprinkle on food.

4. <u>Smoothie Recipes</u>

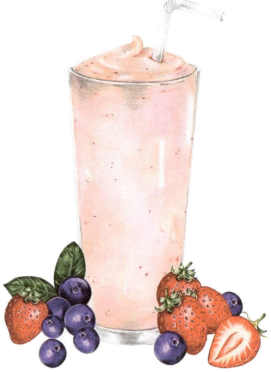

Ingredients:

🩷 **Energy**

- ½ cup dragon fruit or strawberries
- ¼ cup beet juice
- 1 cup almond milk
- 1 scoop protein powder
- 1 tablespoon (tbsp.) hemp seeds

🧡 **Digestion** – help the body process the food you eat

- 1 large carrot
- ½ cup papaya
- 1-inch ginger root
- ½ cup water
- ½ cup coconut water

💛 **Swelling & Bloating**

- ½ cup pineapple
- ½ teaspoon (tsp.) turmeric
- 1 cup nut milk
- 1 tablespoon (tbsp.) chia seeds
- 1 scoop protein powder

Metabolism – help your body use the food you eat

- 1 large handful of kale
- 1/3 cup celery
- 1/3 lemon
- 1 kiwi or green apple
- 1 scoop protein powder
- 1 cup water

 Antioxidants

- ½ cup blueberries
- ½ cup blackberries
- 1 cup nut milk
- 1 scoop protein powder
- 1 tablespoon (tbsp.) hemp seeds

Directions:

- Blend and enjoy.

5. Eat Walnuts

Health Benefits:

- Someone has problems with their skin— a sunburn or they fell and skinned themselves.
- Improve someone's health.
- Someone has cancer.
- Someone wants to have strong bones.
- Someone wants to avoid Diabetes.
- Someone wants to have their body use the food they eat.
- Someone is grumpy.

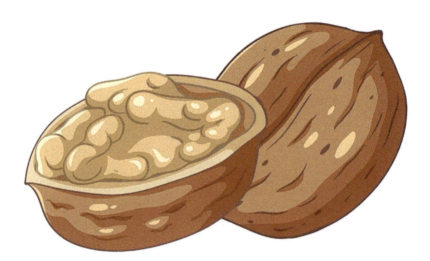

PART 2:
SOMEONE IN MY FAMILY NEEDS HELP

1. **Someone got attacked by a bug**

Recipe:

Mix a little water with activated charcoal (can be purchased as capsules or powder) and apply to:

- bee stings
- snake, ant, spider and wasp bites

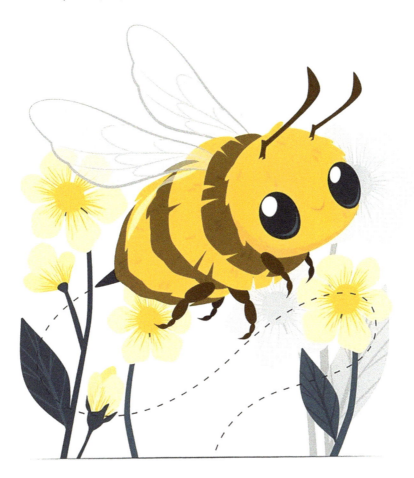

I Can Heal My Family ~ 7

2. Someone Has a Sunburn

Treatment:

- Rub aloe vera, gel or lotion, on the sunburn.
- No aloe?? No worries! Rub a slice of cucumber on the sunburn.

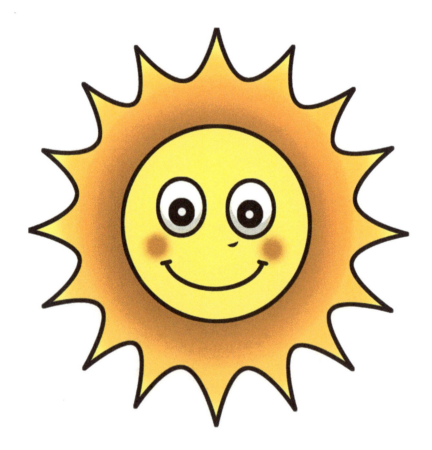

3. Someone I Love Has Cancer

a. Apple and onion

Directions:

- Quarter an apple (including seeds) and onion (including the peel).
- Boil in two cups of water for 10-12 minutes.
- Drink 6oz (1 small glass) 3 times a day.

Onions absorb bacteria. Each serving should be made fresh and drank immediately. It kills bacteria and cancer.

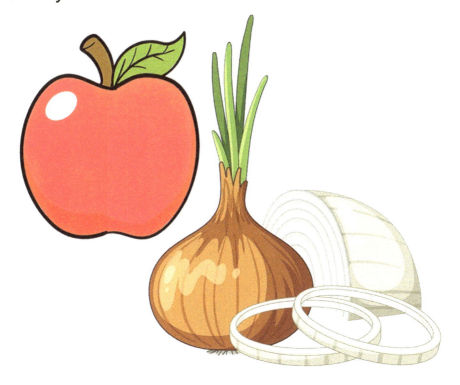

https://www.ncbi.nlm.nih.gov/pmc/articles/PMC442131/

a. **Dandelion Root**

- Able to kill 98% of cancer cells within 48 hours in the laboratory. It is very healthy
- Acts as a powerful anti-inflammatory, immune booster, antioxidant, and organ detoxifier.

Directions:

- Clean and bake roots at 200 degrees for 2 hours.
- Grind or cut up and let sit in hot water to make a tea

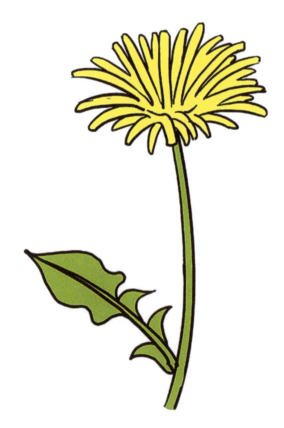

https://www.usatoday.com/story/news/factcheck/2021/ 05/04/ fact-check-dandelion-root-does-not-treat-cancer-two-days/4886361001/

4. Someone Has a Cold

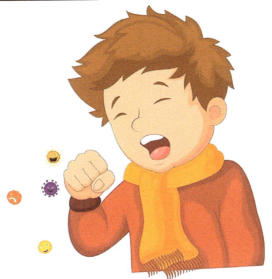

a. **Try this first.**

Ingredients:

- ½ cup of honey
- 1 teaspoon (tsp.) turmeric
- ½ teaspoon (tsp.) ground ginger
- 1 teaspoon (tsp.) vanilla

Directions:

- Mix well and take 1 teaspoon (tsp.) per day.

b. **Cough and Cold Syrup**

Ingredients:

- 1 medium pineapple
- 1 peeled lemon
- 2 inches ginger root

- ½ teaspoon (tsp.) Turmeric
- ½ teaspoon (tsp.) Cayenne pepper
- ¼ teaspoon (tsp.) Black Pepper
- pinch of salt

Directions:

- Blend and drink.

c. **Cough Syrup**

Ingredients:

- ¼ teaspoon (tsp.) cayenne pepper
- ½ teaspoon (tsp.) grated ginger
- ½ teaspoon (tsp.) cinnamon
- 3 tablespoons (tbsp.) raw honey
- 2 tablespoons (tbsp.) apple cider vinegar
- 3 tablespoons (tbsp.) fresh lemon juice
- ½ cup water

Directions:

- Grate the ginger.
- Add all ingredients into a glass jar. Seal it and shake it to mix it together well.
- Store the jar in the refrigerator for up to a week in a sealed container.
- Drink 1 teaspoon (tsp.) at a time and repeat every two hours.

d. **Honey Mixed with Onions**

Directions:

- Chop up onions.
- Pour honey over the onions.
- Leave in a jar. In twelve hours, your syrup will be ready for use.

This is effective against a sore throat.

Take it when you think you are sick or if you have a cough.

Take 1 spoonful once per day until you feel better.

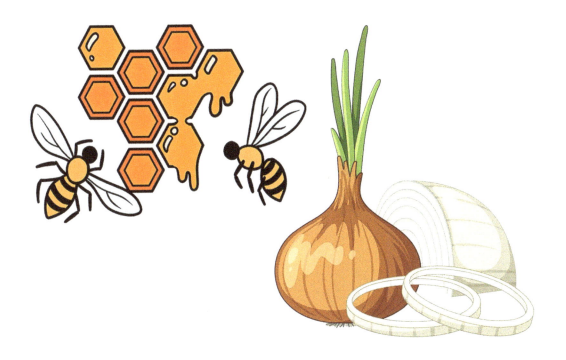

5. Someone Has the Flu

Ingredients:

- ½ cup boiling water
- 1 teaspoon (tsp.) salt
- 1 teaspoon (tsp.) cayenne pepper
- ½ cup apple cider vinegar

Directions:

- Stir water and salt until salt is dissolved.
- Add pepper and vinegar.
- Take 1 tablespoon every 15-20 minutes until the flu symptoms is gone.

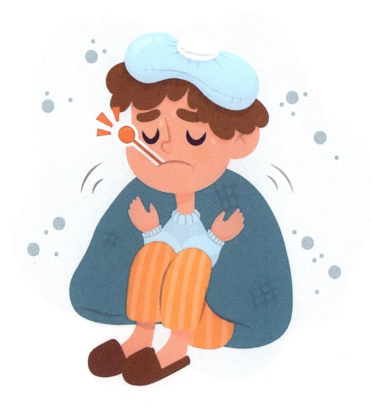

6. Someone Thinks They Are Going to Throw Up

a. Ginger Tea

Ingredients:

- 1-inch piece of ginger root, peeled and sliced into pieces
- 1 cup boiling water
- Honey or lemon juice. (optional)

Directions:

- Put the ginger root piece directly in a mug.
- Add to boiling water and let sit for 5 to 10 minutes.
- Add honey or lemon juice, if desired.

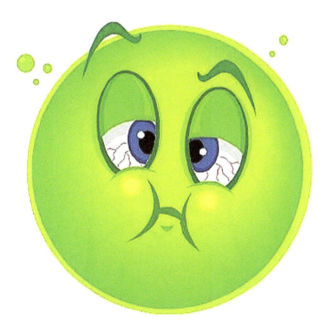

b. **Someone Has a Headache**

Ingredients:

- 4 slices pineapple
- ¼ pound (lb.) turmeric
- ¼ pound (lb.) ginger
- 1 tablespoon (tbsp.) cayenne pepper
- 2 teaspoons (tsp.) black pepper in 12 ounces (oz.) of hot water

Directions:

- Blend and strain,
- Store in refrigerator in airtight container.
- 6 teaspoons (tsp.) twice a day.
- Children over the age of one can add in honey.

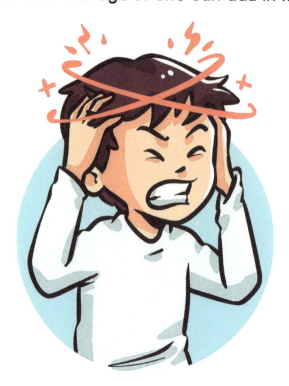

c. **Someone Has a Toothache**

Ingredients:

- clove oil
- coconut oil
- turmeric
- garlic

Directions:

- Mix equal parts clove oil and coconut oil with a 1/8 teaspoon (tsp.) of turmeric.
- Swish in mouth and spit it out.
- Repeat as needed.

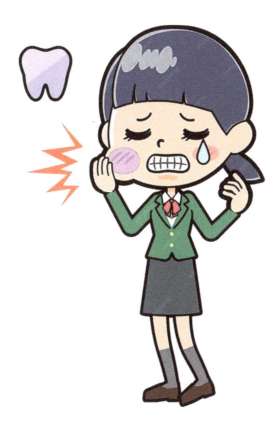

Conclusion

My hope is that you find something in these pages to help you achieve better health for yourself and your family.

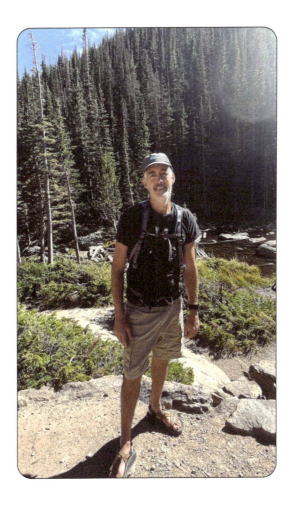

Sources

1. Front page illustration : https://easydrawingguides.com/how-to-draw-a-family/

2. Honey illustration: https://easydrawingguides.com/how-to-draw-a-honeycomb/

3. Lemon illustration : https://easydrawingguides.com/how-to-draw-a-lemon/

4. Lemon peel illustration: https://www.shutterstock.com/search/lemon-peel?page=2 - Lemon Peel royalty-free image

5. Smoothie illustration: https://www.freepik.com/free-vector/illustration-fruit-smoothie-drink-watercolor-style_2782930.htm#page=2&query=smoothie&position=9&from_view=search&track=sph&uuid=d408dce7-d0c7-4ce0-90d7-7a2af830b5b3

6. Walnuts illustration : https://www.freepik.com/free-vector/isolated-simple-walnut-cartoon_38346876.htm#query=walnuts&position=29&from_view=search&track=sph&uuid=3329b2e4-f7d6-4195-b72e-427611ec15b7

7. Bee illustration : https://www.freepik.com/free-vector/bee-concept-illustration_42107949.htm#query=bee&position=40&from_view=search&track=sph&uuid=8c514c75-0fd3-4175-ba56-a5d82acfeaae

8. Sun illustration : http://drawdoo.com/draw/sun/

9. Apple illustration : https://iheartcraftythings.com/apple-drawing.html

10. Onion illustration : https://www.freepik.com/free-vector/isolated-onion-cartoon-style_39264687.htm#query=onion&position=3&from_view=search&track=sph&uuid=28db340e-7496-4732-8002-8ac63f5fd6b6

11. Flu illustration : https://www.freepik.com/free-vector/person-with-cold-thermometer_7334440.htm#page=3&query=flu%20drawing&position=34&from_view=search&track=ais&uuid=fceca333-f932-4697-a060-6d03dc5008c3

12. Nauseous illustration: https://img.freepik.com/free-vector/puke-emoji_53876-25520.jpg?t=st=1706292025~exp=1706292625~hmac=2c13c2da3f768502e63800c9e839852b02b9460d76e721a21da5b7c6e8188047

I Can Heal My Family ~ 21

13. Headache illustration: https://www.freepik.com/free-vector/hand-drawn-headache-cartoon-illustration_59741414.htm#query=headache%20drawing&position=2&from_view=search&track=ais&uuid=89c20529-e9e3-48d8-b8fc-3a99ae5bc29c

14. Toothache illustration: https://www.freepik.com/premium-vector/out-line-school-girl-green-musiba_8552426.htm#page=2&query=toothache%20cartoon&position=6&from_view=search&track=ais&uuid=54ea9f7a-1698-4f08-9498-8ee6b6f3b217

www.ingramcontent.com/pod-product-compliance
Ingram Content Group UK Ltd.
Pitfield, Milton Keynes, MK11 3LW, UK
UKHW050716131224
452350UK00027B/139